IF YOU KNEW HOW REGULAR I AM… YOU WOULDN'T BE SO FULL OF IT

*My 30 Year Secret Life
With Crohn's Disease*

by

Toni Whitley

Bloomington, IN  Milton Keynes, UK

authorHOUSE®

AuthorHouse™
1663 Liberty Drive, Suite 200
Bloomington, IN 47403
www.authorhouse.com
Phone: 1-800-839-8640

AuthorHouse™ UK Ltd.
500 Avebury Boulevard
Central Milton Keynes, MK9 2BE
www.authorhouse.co.uk
Phone: 08001974150

First published by AuthorHouse 4/14/2007

ISBN: 978-1-4259-9659-8 (sc)

Printed in the United States of America
Bloomington, Indiana

This book is printed on acid-free paper.

"Your book was very informative concerning the intricacies of Crohn's Disease. Your attention to detail in explaining your emotions and concerns was heartfelt. I believe your book would be a welcome addition to a person who is afflicted with this disease and their family and friends to help cope with their situations. God Bless and the best of luck."

Andrea Bragg, Executive Assistant
Office Of Congresswoman Carolyn C.. Kilpatrick

"Your description of your on-going battle with this debilitating disease is a real eye-opener. You bring to life the difficulties you have endured in trying to do the things the rest of us take for granted."

Karen Sovel
Disability Benefits Service, PLLC

"Reading upon the struggles and challenges that you've faced, you've applied the wisdom and teachings of what you've learned by parents and your pastor to get you through some of the toughest of times. Even though you had ongoing infirmities in your body, you didn't stay down and let it overtake you, but you've endured it, overcame your fears and continued to reach your goals."

Sister Sandra Crump
Door of Faith Ministries

Acknowledgements

I'd like to acknowledge and thank the following persons for their continued support and/or input in my completing this project at a time when I was at the lowest point of my life.

With their continued prayers and encouragement, I was able to regain the strength and motivation to complete this book.

First and foremost, I'd like to Thank God. For He has sustained me and given me mercy.

Through his mercy, I have been delivered from the insanity that my most recent ordeal had me going through. And for that, I give him continued praise.

I'd like to thank my long-time friend and personal photographer, John Evans, of Akron, OH.

Thank you, John, for putting up with me as I was going through and also, for your artistic advice on this bookcover.

One of the advantages of having a 'root' in your life, is that their friendship is steadfast. And that is what I have found in my relationship with my puberty girlfriend, Gloria Ford (GiGi) of Oakland, CA. Thank you for your pointing me into this direction. While in the midst of my insanity, GiGi dropped everything and came out to see about me, not once, but twice during this period. To keep me busy and my mind occupied, I began working with her on her upcoming book, "Don't Lose Your Clients Because They're Losing Their Hair". By working on her project, she encouraged and inspired me to write my own story.

Lastly, I'd like to thank my pastor, Rev. Earl O. Crump, of Door of Faith in Pontiac, MI for his many prayers and his understanding. Having been an active member of his church since 2000, it was very hard for me to recently discuss with him what I have been going through with this disease.

But I felt that he needed to know why I was no longer attending church services on a regular basis. Thank you, Rev. Crump for the tapes you gave me to listen to during this period.

INSPIRATION

This book is comprised of my personal 30 year struggle with Crohn's Disease. During the past year, my condition has deteriorated to its lowest point ever. Not only has my medical condition gone to an all time low; but emotionally—I feel as though I've just been delivered from an "out of mind" experience which had made me feel on some days that I'd never regain my mind back. Emotional and mood swings are so closely associated with this disorder that stressful situations can take you overboard.

My personal situation of stress being taken overboard has been a continuous fight with the insurance carrier and social security disability to acknowledge this chronic disorder as such; learning how to discuss my disorder with others without breaking down crying; and most importantly having to continue to make my son feel secure and loved no matter what I'm going through. After keeping this disorder a secret from friends and family for so many years; I have recently gotten better at expressing myself due to the treatment of depression with a therapist over the past several months.

To my chagrin, however, it has really surprised me how little anyone knows about this disorder. Even though there are over 500,000 people in America affected with Crohn's Disease, it seems to be a "little kept secret" by many others. Unlike cancer, diabetes, and other such chronic illnesses there is very little, if any media coverage on this disorder. Daytime talk shows are generally the platform to discuss a variety of health topics; but unfortunately none of these shows have covered this topic to the full extent of the challenges that crohn's sufferers deal with on a daily basis. While doing research on-line for various support groups (Healingwell.com and Crohn's Zone.com) to help me deal better with this disease, these disturbing facts seems to be the normal concerns of thousands of sufferers:

There are thousands of young people in their late teens and early 20's that have recently been diagnosed with this disorder. They are feeling as if their lives have already ended because they lack the courage it takes to meet the daily challenges of living with this disease;

Although surgery is not a cure, based on information from these various support groups show that there seems to be a lot of people having multiple surgeries, yet they are still suffering from physical and emotional problems;

Since there has been very little advancement in the treatment or cure of this disease, there are many people struggling financially because they are being dropped by insurance carriers and denied disability at an alarming rate. Many of these sufferers are facing a life-long disorder with severe symptoms but they are expected to pretend to fit into society's high esteem on appearances; and

Lastly, my own personal concern is the majority of the sufferers posted on these support groups usually have their pictures next to their names and I have yet to see someone that looks like me (African-American female).

After countless hours of praying; listening to spiritual tapes and hearing the "Word" from my pastor, I have decided to write this book; not only for the young people that are suffering from a life-long disorder (of any kind), but am attempting to inspire anyone that need a story (testimony) to encourage them and give them hope that their dreams do not have to be forgotten because of a diagnoses or because of where they come from.

Yesterday, I Cried

I cried because I hurt. I cried because I was hurt. I cried because hurt has no place to go except deeper into the pain that caused it in the first place, and when it gets there, the hurt wakes you up. I cried because it was too late. I cried because it was time. I cried because my soul knew that I didn't know that my soul knew everything I needed to know. I cried a soulful cry yesterday, and it felt so good. It felt so very, very bad. In the midst of my crying I felt my freedom coming, because YESTERDAY, I CRIED WITH AN AGENDA..

(Taken from *Yesterday, I Cried* by Iylana Vanzant)

INTRODUCTION

If someone would have asked me a year ago to describe myself to them, I would have responded something like this:

> "My name is Toni. I am a 51 year old successful, African-American woman and single mom to a 12-year old son. Over the past 30 years working for corporate America, I am currently a Financial Planning Consultant for a large corporation that I've worked for over 20 years (in three different states). My favorite pastime is shopping, going to cultural events and eating out. And would also tell them that I am a Christian and believe that God has been there for me when I wasn't there for myself."
>
> I would have told them almost everything they wanted to know about me except for my 30 year secret. My secret is I have had an almost

30 year battle with Crohn's Disease. You may ask, "Why would you keep that a secret?" Well, I would have to take you back 30 years ago when I was initially diagnosed with this disorder. My then elderly physician (with the bedside manners of Hannibal) explained the disorder to me and then ended the conversation by telling me that Irritable Bowel Disorders (IBD) was a 'shameful' disease and most people do not talk about it. They keep the disorder to themselves. And henceforth, that was the only thing that stuck in my mind for years. My determination to succeed in life was my top priority so I chose to keep this to myself and continue to grow educationally and professionally. I also continued to hold on to the dream of becoming a model.

What is Crohn's Disease? Crohn's Disease is a chronic inflammatory disease of the intestines. It primarily causes ulcerations (breaks in the lining) of the small and large intestines, but can affect the digestive system anywhere from the mouth to the anus. Symptoms include stomach cramps and pain that comes and goes, diarrhea and blood in the stool, weight lost; nausea and vomiting; as well as fatigue and joint pains. While some people have severe symptoms, some may have less severe symptoms. Some people who have the disease have long periods without any symptoms (even without getting treatments). Others with more severe disease will need long-term treatment or even surgery.

Its name was derived from Dr. Crohn, a physician who described the disease back in 1932. It is also called glaucomatous enteritis or colitis, regional enteritis, ileitis, or terminal ileitis. Crohn's Disease is closely related to another chronic inflammatory disorder called Ulcerative Colitis. They are both frequently referred to as Irritable Bowel Disorders. They are both chronic conditions which dramatically impacts the sufferer's quality of life. Since they both can involve uncontrollable diarrhea, severe abdominal pain and nausea, not only does it make employment difficult but it also makes it difficult to discuss these symptoms with others.

Because their symptoms are so closely related, throughout the years, depending on the physician diagnosing my symptoms, I have received both diagnoses as my disorder. Neither one has a medical cure. Once the disease begins, they tend to fluctuate between periods of inactivity (remission) and activity (relapse). They affect approximately one-half to two million people in the U.S. They are most common among women, Caucasians and Jewish people. The cause is unknown but neither disease is contagious. Although diet may affect the symptoms, it is unlikely the source of the disease. Latest research suggests that they may be caused by a malfunction in the body's immune system. Certain environmental factors may also increase the risk for Irritable Bowel Disorders. It seems to run in families but there is no known pattern of inheritance. In my case, my father has suffered with intestinal disorders, such as ulcers. On my mother's side of the family, I am told that her grandmother died unexpectedly from "Acute Indigestion".

The treatment varies depending on the severity of the disease. In my case, I have been on the same medications for so many years that they are no longer effective. I've been on the anti-inflammatory medications (such as Sulfasalazine). Steroids and cortisone are frequently used for treatment (such as Prednisone); but they really take me on an emotional rollercoaster. There have been times throughout the years when I'd be in public (at work, social events, family gatherings, etc.) when my mood would change with the blink of an eye. I could be joyful one minute and the next in tears. Not only does the Prednisone give you major mood swings, but it also bloats you. It's commonly known as the "moon face" drug among colitis and crohn's patients. With all the downsides of Prednisone, I would have to admit that it would put my relapses back under control. In recent months, since my last relapse, I have been taking a newer medication called Infliximab (brand name Remicade). These are infusion treatments that are used in severe cases.

The other alternative is surgery which at this time I am totally against due to the fact that there is no surgical cure. Even when all of the parts of the diseased parts of the intestines are removed, inflammation frequently reoccurs in previously healthy intestines months to years after the surgery. About 50% of patients can expect a reoccurrence of symptoms within four years of surgery.

Depression and other mood disorders are very closely associated with Crohn's Disease. I am sure that it is due to the stress that you are constantly under. The stress may result from the challenges of daily routines. Especially for those that are trying to hold down a full-time job. Because of the symptoms, it is very difficult to plan your day out in advance, due to the fact that each day your symptoms may vary from mild to extreme, without warning. Also, the stress of trying to hide the fact you're suffering from this awful disease can compound matters. Well, in my case it was stressful trying to hide the fact that there was this awful medical problem that I have been living with since the age of 22.

Contents

CHAPTER ONE
FINALLY, ON MY OWN

Coming from a background of being poor, African-American and female, growing up in the 60's, you were constantly given the unwanted message from others (being family, teachers, or media) of your limitations in life. Even my loving mother (in her naivety) saw success as marrying a "good hard working man" that loved you deeply was pretty much all you needed. It didn't matter if you had dreams of your own. Having desires to branch out into the world all alone was unheard of in my family. It may have resulted from the fact that my mother had lived in one state her entire life. She went straight from high school to marriage to motherhood. That was what she knew and that was what made her happy. I didn't see my future taking that course, however. I don't remember the exact day or whether it was someone I heard on television, or a school teacher or whomever. I don't remember the exact words that it was. All I know is that I became aware of this wonderful world outside of my environment and I just had to become a part of it.

As early as I can remember, having been born in Detroit and raised in the small town of Saginaw, MI; my dream was to finish high school and move to New York to become a model. My mother, Shirlene (she still lives in Saginaw) was a very beautiful woman. She was very well built, but petite. She wore her makeup impeccably (in the 50's and 60's) before makeup was cool. I would love to watch her dress up to go out. Her face was a pure piece of beauty once she arched her eyebrows and put on the different shades of eyeshadow. Sometimes for a more dramatic affect, she would put on false eyelashes. Her skin was flawless. She was constantly getting compliments on how well she dressed and how pretty she was.

She put so much pride into looking great at all times and she also put the same pride into dressing me and my older sister, Marshon. She never wanted us to dress in the trendy fashions, but wanted us to look different. We hated it at the time. My sister and I always complained that we dressed so different from the other kids. Even our hairdos were way out at times. She would experiment with different hairdos (mostly to hide the burns from the straightening comb on our ears and neck). But as much as my sister and I complained, the more compliments we received from the other kids at school. They actually liked the way we dressed. They said we were "sharp".

By the time I finished high school, I still harbored the desire to leave Michigan. After reluctantly attending community college for a couple of semesters; with the aide of my step-father, we were finally able to convince my mother to allow me to leave home. With the proceeds from the sale of my Ford Maverick, I paid off my two small credit card accounts and began making plans to move. We agreed on my moving to Linden, New Jersey (a small town outside of Newark). On August 10, 1975, we stood in our garage with my mother crying her goodbyes as my stepfather and I loaded the car with my luggage. Within a half hour later, I boarded the Greyhound Bus with all of my worldly possessions (clothes, hats, shoes and books).

After moving in with my step-father's brother and his family (Johnny and Lula Rozier), they immediately put me to work at their neighborhood candy store. My uncles Johnny and Charlie owned the store and they only paid me about $1 to $2 an hour and expected me to work 40 hours a week. Today kids would think they were crazy and refuse to do it, but I worked for them to show my appreciation for all they were doing for me.

Linden was a very small town with a lot of Carolinians. It was very much like Saginaw. Everybody knows everybody kind-of-town. African-Americans lived on one side of town and the Caucasians on the other. It didn't take me long to adjust to my new home. I was meeting a lot of people while working at the store. Since I had grown up in a Baptist church back home, I joined one of the neighborhood Baptist churches out of tradition and was one of those 11am Sunday morning only members.

I learned my way around town within a week because like most small towns, there was one main street that could take you anywhere you needed to go. In Linden, that street was St. George's Avenue which if I went south, I'd be in Rahway and north would take me to Elizabeth. It took me about two weeks to learn the freeways.

Once I enrolled in a secretarial school (Sawyer School, Inc.), I was put on the work study program and was able to gain part-time employment at an engineering firm in Newark. With my heavy schedule of going to school; working at the engineering firm and then ending the evening at the store (which stayed open until 10 or 11pm); I'd have to admit that my eating habits had changed tremendously. For the first time ever, I was eating a lot at fast food restaurants for breakfast and lunch. And because my income was so limited, most days I could only afford to go to White Castles which was across the street from the engineering firm. To this date, I cannot stand to look at a White Castles. It brings back bad memories of eating their $2 value lunch almost on a daily basis.

Between my two uncles, they provided me with a car to drive to and from school and work everyday. Prior to my getting the part-time job in Newark, I had to catch the bus to school everyday. There was about a five or six block walk from where I lived to the bus stop. I was fortunate because whenever the weather was bad, I'd get a ride from the bus stop by a passerby that knew me from the store. I wouldn't recommend this habit to a young person today because things are so much different today. Back in the day, you just trusted people more to do the right thing.

In May 1976, I received my certificate for a Professional Secretary from Sawyers (it only took me six months to complete the nine month course) and immediately began receiving job referrals from the school to various companies in New Jersey and New York. I was praying for a job in New York but my first full-time job offer was from an agency in Newark.

By August 1976, I was hired on as a stenographer-secretary at United Community Corporation (UCC) which is one of the few anti-poverty agencies still in existence today. I worked for the Director of the Head Start Programs in Newark. I liked the job because it gave me a lot of experience of working in the field, meeting with city officials and politicians. Ken Gibson (who was the first African-American Mayor elected in a major city) was the mayor at that time. At least once or twice a month, we held board meetings which would include city officials, as well as board members of UCC and Head Start. The meetings would last from two hours or more and it was my responsibility to take extensive minutes of what was discussed at these meetings. I did not have the privilege of using a dictaphone machine or tape recorder back then. Therefore; I had to rely on Gregg Shorthand skills to get the job done.

After being on the job for a few months, I began my search for an apartment in Newark. Since I was single and this was my first apartment, security was a huge concern for me. New Hope Village was a fairly new apartment complex which provided 24-hour security;

a laundry room in the building and it was centrally located about 2 miles from my job on Central Avenue and only a couple of miles to Essex College and Rutgers University. It was also only a few miles from downtown Newark. The new Medical/Dentistry Center was being constructed right across the street from the complex and it was an up and coming section of Newark that everyone was interested in. Initially, when I went to the leasing office to apply for an apartment there, I was told that there was a very long waiting list to get an apartment. After informing my new boss of this, he made a phone call to city hall and my name was moved to the top immediately. I applied for an apartment the beginning of the week and was approved for move in only a few days later. This is when I learned the old adage; 'it's not what you know; but who you know' was really true.

Once situated in my new apartment, I enrolled at Essex County College and later transferred to Rutgers University. Both were within walking distance. Looking back to those days, I did a lot of walking. Weather permitting; I walked to and from work, as well as to school. When the weather was bad or if I just didn't feel like walking; there was the bus stop right across the street from me. The mass transportation worked out well for me since my income was too small to afford a car at the time.

My first year at UCC was uneventful (medically). I was happy with my job and decorating my apartment. Unlike most people on a small budget, I quickly went into debt purchasing wall-to-wall carpet, having mirrors and wallpaper installed (and I was only renting). I had a beautiful apartment but was highly leveraged in credit card debt. I had never had to budget before then and had not been taught about financial planning on any level. That was because my parents lived from paycheck-to-paycheck. I was so naïve that I never realized when I lived at home that we were poor. Because we never missed a meal, dressed nice and went on vacations every year, I thought we were at least middle-classed. (Ha-ha-ha).

In 1977, I began having stomach problems. I would get nauseated quite often. I was told by a co-worker once that if I ate salt, it would take away the nausea feeling. I tried eating some salt and miraculously it worked. That was the beginning of my newly found obsession with salt. I kept the little packets of salt in my desk drawer for emergencies. Later, in addition to the nausea, I began having to run to the bathroom more throughout the day. Some days I would suffer from constipation and others diarrhea. They were mostly always accompanied with stomach cramps. After finally going to the doctor for an exam, I was informed that I had Colitis and was given some medications to control the symptoms.

In the midst of the beginning of an illness which would linger on; I still had a life to live. I tried very hard not to let this be a setback for me. I continued working hard everyday; as well as take classes in Business Administration. Since I didn't know anyone in Newark when I first moved there, I was also beginning to meet friends which later became my surrogate family. We would hang out in New York on the weekends, going to broadway plays, shopping, eating out and of course disco partying. Our favorite disco spots in NY were Leviticus and the Cellar. One night we were even invited to Soho to be part of the party people on one of Kurtis Blow's albums. That was very exciting because at the time, he was one of the first rappers on the scene. And it was a pleasure to meet him and see that he was such a 'regular homeboy.'

When I wasn't feeling bad, I always liked to entertain at home. It was in Newark that I began my annual tradition of hosting the Thanksgiving dinner which I continue to do today. I also would frequently throw parties which always turned out great. My friends would come from different cities within New Jersey; as well as New York. There were never any confrontations or arguments; only good food and good times. I was really enjoying my new life in the big city and was growing into a self-sufficient, respectable young lady.

Early spring of 1978, after a brief hospitalization with my illness; it wasn't but a short time later that I left UCC under unpleasant circumstances. However, looking back over my experiences, I now realize that this was a pivotal experience for me. Working for a Black corporation really prepared me for the White corporate America that I would go to in later years. I now had a back-bone and was ready to begin my climb up the corporate ladder.

SUMMATION:
TOOLS I USED DURING
THESE TIMES...

Life is a never-ending journey of learning. Since I had chosen to leave home and embark on a new life in a strange place surrounded by people that knew very little or nothing about me, I quickly realized that I needed tools more than I needed people. The initial tools that would sustain me on my new journey were: sacrifice; independence; reliability; resourcefulness and interchangeability.

SACRIFICE: Right from the onset of my journey, I realized that sacrifice would be a major part of my new lifestyle. Coming from a poor family, you learned at an early age how to differentiate between necessity and discretionary expenses. You had to make choices. Do I spend my last dollar on getting my hair done or pay my phone bill? Well, you begin to make choices that may sometimes turn out to have been a bad choice; but being that you learn from your mistakes, the next time you are in the same situation you are better prepared to make a wiser decision. So when you live on a limited income, you learn how to stretch a dollar. You realize that you can't give in to many temptations and learn to put them on hold until a better day.

Being that I grew up in a family (the major state for automotive industry), I was always surrounded with nice cars. Dad, step-dad, grandparents, uncles, everyone had nice cars. By the time I was 13, I was driving Cadillacs and Buicks. Since I had grown up in an atmosphere where pretty cars were always available to me; I wasn't hung up or impressed by other people's cars. Therefore, it was easy for me to sacrifice not owning a car and using mass transportation and my feet for such a long period of time.

RELIABILITY: I knew that I had to be reliable to maintain a job, as well as being able to build on personal relationships. Reliability is the characteristic which helps you measure a person's loyalty. Therefore, during the early years of my journey, I was very intent on being reliable. And I expected the same from others. Since I measured my reliability towards others, this characteristic taught me to always take care of my personal business for myself. No matter what I was going through medically, I had to make sure that I wrote out my checks to pay my bills on time.

INDEPENDENCE: With my newfound life away from the guardianship of parents, it gave me the freedom to explore without limitations. This freedom was profound. There are so many things available to you in the world and only you can limit yourself through the eyes of others telling you what you can or cannot achieve. If you treasure your independence, you will not let what others say hold you back. And the ironic thing is that most of the time, the ones that are trying to place the limitations on you, have not even attempted to 'step outside of their own box'. The freedom to make your own choices and then began to implement them, are invaluable. You can set your own goals and no one but yourself can hold you back once you fully declare yourself as being independent.

RESOURCEFULNESS: I will tell you one thing. You will need this tool to give you the ability to handle any unforeseen situations that may arise. For me, it started off with small things; such as if I only have $20 left after paying rent and all of my other essential expenses, how am I going to eat for the next two weeks when my next paycheck comes in? Well, one good thing about growing up poor, not only do you learn how to stretch a dollar, but you also learn how to stretch food. By the time I was 12 years old, I could prepare about 10 different meals out of hamburger meat. And not only that, I could stretch the meat with cracker crumbs. So in my new journey, it was easy for me to go grocery shopping on Mulberry Street and pick up some fresh vegetables and go to the butcher shop and get so many pounds of hamburger, oxtails and turkey wings. You'd be surprised how many meals I could prepare from maybe spending $10 to $20 on groceries (and had coupons for mostly everything). If I ran out of food prior to payday, then I'd open a can of soup. Oh, and let me not forget to tell you my story about the pantyhose. If I had a run in one leg of my pantyhose, I'd cut off the good leg of two pairs and turn them into one pair. Now that was being resourceful. I think that this was the characteristic that kept me from going into the 'shallow' realm of life. It kept me grounded and reminded me of where I came from.

INTERCHANGEABILITY: The tool of knowing when something or some-one should be substituted or replaced. People that come into your life are interchangeable and that is a good thing. It is only a bad thing when we don't realize it. Now that I have learned that people are like seasons: they will come and go; it is very important to differentiate when their season has ended. No one explains it better than Tyler Perry when he makes his dissertation of people in your life compared to a tree. Most people are like leaves and we have to know when they are passing through our lives and when to let them go. A few others may be like a branch, remain in our lives but will sway. But if we are fortunate enough to find someone that is like a root; we should hold on to that one because the root will be steadfast and always in your corner. I have found that I have had many leaves and branches, but not many roots. But do you really need many roots?

I can even break this interchangeability into another phase of my life that I have learned over the years. Classic will always outweigh trends. I have learned that if I go with the classic style, I can turn one outfit into several (with changing up accessories) and hold on to that one suit (weight permitting) for years. The same principle applies to buying furniture. If you buy quality and classic the first time; reupholstery can take you a long way.

Chapter Two
My Attempt at Boldness
(New York---Here I am)

Over the years, it has been my personal experience that change can be good. I turned out to be a person that would take chances and explore my options. I knew my time was about to run its course at UCC so I set out to look for a job in New York. With resume' in hand, I started interviewing with various companies in New York. It was exhilarating to me just to have the opportunity to run around the city interviewing at various top-notch ad agencies, law firms, etc. Whomever I heard were hiring, I was there with my resume'. Keeping in mind that this was also during the time of the notorious days of "The Son of Sam" killing single women; my mother had more fear about it than me. I was on a mission and wouldn't be stopped. Hanging out in the city until night and taking the commute back to Newark without a care in the world was a thrilling experience to me. The possibility of being in an area where there were so many opportunities and my being exposed to them (merely by being at the right place at the right time) was an adventure. That thought alone is what kept me going. Because in all honesty, when I look back today, I don't know how I did it. Walking through the different stations; rushing to catch a train or bus. I had to pretend not to be closely watching the crazies sitting on the subway off into their la-la world. I'd sit on the subway with that look on my face which I had practiced over-and-over again. The look which implied, "Hey, I'm crazy too so don't even think about messing with me."

All of the interviews finally paid off and I nabbed a job in New York City. It was a dream come true. I was hired on at MacMillan Publishing Company on Third Avenue and 53rd Street. It was hard to believe that I was now working in the heart of Manhattan. I was hired on as a statistical secretary to the Comptroller of the company. He was a very distinguished looking, well-dressed gentleman. Sort of like a white-haired, older Regis Philbin. He was also very old school. I had to work on a manual typewriter. But it was okay. Just the excitement of working in New York was the main thing.

Although I still lived in Newark, the test of my endurance was my personal challenge and I was ready for it. I would dress as sharp as I could everyday and walk outside to the corner bus stop for my ride from W. Market Street to downtown Newark. Once I got off at

Newark's Penn Station, I would take the first mode of transportation leaving for New York. The bus departing from the station would take me to Port Authority on 42nd Street; the Amtrak train would let me off at Grand Central Station; or if I took the Path Train, it would take me to the World Trade Center. Which ever source got me into New York, I'd take the subway to my final destination to work. Either route was euphoric for a country girl from very humble beginnings.

I learned the shopping game in New York very quickly. It was about looking great without paying too much. The garment district and Orchard Street (off Canal Street) was well known for great bargains. On Orchard Street, you could negotiate your price at most of the stores. That is where I purchased my first fox coat at a very low price. I would stand on the subway track in the winter with my fox and sharp outfit (with matching hat of course) waiting on the train looking good.

I must admit that working in New York has been one of the most thrilling experiences of my life, so far. The smell of the city, the noise, as well as the hustle and bustle is something that can only be experienced there. The plays, restaurants and the fashion capital of the world; simply said, 'there's no place like New York'. People have always said that New Yorkers are the most unfriendly people. I found that to be totally untrue. Usually, being the stranger or new face in the place; the people that I would encounter always welcomed me as if they'd known me forever. Yes, I was enjoying every aspect of working in New York.

I was so enthralled with the experience that it caught me off guard when I relapsed and had to go out on sick leave. Again, the 'colitis' was acting up. (In 1977, I had this problem and was diagnosed with colitis and given some Alzulphadine and Prednisone. (The medications seemed to have corrected the problem, so I thought.) This time, I was given the same prescriptions and returned to my normal routine. The large high-rise office building I worked in had a full cafeteria downstairs so instead of running out to different restaurants or to the corner hotdog stands, I was able to discipline myself to pack a bland lunch on most days, in an attempt to improve my diet. Initially, diet seemed to make a significant difference in how active the symptoms would affect me.

Now that I was feeling better, I began working on a photo portfolio so I could get my goal of modeling back on track. On the weekends, I began working on the photos to submit to Ford and Wilhelmina Modeling Agencies in New York. I was feeling great again and was rejuvenated.

On my payday, I normally stopped to buy something for myself on the way home. My favorite shopping spot in the World Trade Center was the Plymouth. It was an affordable boutique which sold women's clothing and accessories. They also sold nice looking hats. If I were happy, I'd buy a hat; if I were depressed, I'd buy a hat. I just bought hats. Any excuse. Over the years, I probably have had several hundred hats.

I didn't stay in remission long this time. My body was beginning to really feel the effects of this disease on a more regular basis. Now imagine this, if you can (my typical day with this disorder and commuting to New York from Newark). I would leave home to catch the bus or train into New York. I would pray that the urge to go to the restroom before I could catch a bus or train from Newark would not overtake me. Then I said another prayer while on the way to New York not to have the urge to defecate. Then the times began increasing when I would have to get off the train and run to the restroom prior to boarding the subway. I must have known where every public restroom was between Newark and New York. It became a normal part of my commute. During the times of relapses, the nausea and cramps were added to the symptoms as well.

By September 1979, I was sick again. Maybe it was denial, but initially I told myself I had the stomach flu. After a couple of days staying in bed, balled up in pain from stomach cramps and not being able to hold anything on my stomach, I finally decided to go back to the doctor. With my loyal surrogate family coming over bringing me soups and juices for a few days, I was finally convinced that it wasn't just a flu bug but maybe related to the similar problem of colitis. Since colitis wasn't a well known disorder back then, I guess I didn't realize the seriousness of the condition. And because the term Irritable Bowel Disorder still sounded so offensive to me; I remained quiet about it to my family and friends.

By the time my dehydrated body made it to the doctor's office, he was ready to hospitalize me for some tests to determine if my condition was colitis or crohn's. The tests they gave back then to determine whether or not you were affected with IBD were just as bad as the disorder itself. The first test I remember having to take was the barium enema test. I had to drink about a quart of this chalky flavored white substance that tasted horrible. It made me gag each time I attempted to swallow it. But they forced me to drink it all in order for them to perform the test they had to take. Then came the good old sigmoidoscopy" and 'colonoscopy' procedures. The preparation for these tests was just as bad as the test themselves. I had to drink a gallon of liquid that also made me gag. I could not eat anything for a day prior to the actual tests. And the worse part was that back then, they would not put you to sleep for these tests. You had to be wide awake. I CAN'T EVEN BEGIN TO DESCRIBE THE PAIN INFLICTED BY THESE TESTS. Once while having the sigmoidoscopy test, I was in so much pain that I actually pulled my weave out of my hair during the procedure. I am so thankful that over the years, these tests have become painless. Now you are put to sleep for the procedure and do not feel a thing. The preparation for the tests is the most uncomfortable part.

This time the results came back with the diagnoses of "Ulcerative Colitis" which is a more severe case of colitis. I was also diagnosed with severe anemia. After remaining in the hospital for over two weeks, I was released with the instructions to remain on the Prednisone and Alzulphadine. The doctor prescribed B12 shots for the anemia and to boost my energy level. Going back on the bland diet was also recommended. Over the years, I was put on a bland diet so much that it has become my normal way of eating.

Unfortunately, those that have suffered from this disease will know how I felt when I returned to work and was told that my job was no longer available to me. My hospitalization stay was from 9/16 thru 10/4 and that did not include the additional week or two that I had to remain off from work to recuperate. I was told that my position had to be filled but they would contact me if another position were to become open. It is a known fact that most people do not understand this disorder and do not realize that it is a chronic disease. However, insurance companies as well as social security disability does not see it as such and there are many of those (us) that are left without medical coverage or are dropped from insurance coverage due to the disorder. It is a necessity for us to have insurance because the health care costs are so astronomical that we cannot afford to pay for our care without coverage. Therefore, I knew that I had no other choice but to find another job immediately. I could not wait for MacMillan Publishing to call me back (as if they were going to call back an employee with a pre-existing medical condition).

Therefore, I decided to go to the temporary agencies for quick placement. Manpower and Kelly Services were good at placing you into a temporary job expediently. I figured this would provide me with some temporary funds while I looked for something permanent. Besides, I was still young and not financially astute. I had a little savings account but not enough to cover my rent for the month. So this was an emergency. It was my determination since leaving home not to have to call home and ask for financial assistance from my family so I had to make the temporary agency work for me. I refused to make my family think I couldn't make it on my own.

While working that winter for the temporary agency, I happened upon LeSecretaire, an agency which only specialized in hiring legal secretaries. It was ideal for me. It was freelance secretarial work which paid more than I had made on any of my previous jobs. I was free to work at my discretion and I was also able to pay into a health-care plan which I could afford. It was another ideal job. However, it wasn't in New York. Most of my job assignments were in Central New Jersey, working for the major law firms as a legal secretary. The assignments usually lasted three to four months at a time. Since I was good at what I was doing, I usually requested back by the same law firms when they needed a temp. That was good for me because on the repeat assignments, I would be familiar with their office procedures. I was receiving job offers at most of the law firms but was enjoying this flexibility so much that I would not accept any of the offers to go permanent. As a matter of fact, after about a year of doing this temporary work, I began my own schedule. I would work an assignment (usually three to four months) then I'd go on a vacation. This is when I began to travel.

I had friends in California (Los Angeles, San Mateo, and Oakland), Chicago, Atlanta, and New Orleans and would get on a plane and go. Back in the 70's and 80's, flying was glamorous. I'd dress up and get on the plane and feel like I was a star. There is no glamour in flying anymore. But I was having the time of my life.....in between the relapses.

Another good thing about working the temporary agencies is that I now was forced to buy a car. Since my job assignments were in Morristown, Basking Ridge, the Oranges, as well as downtown Newark, I no longer was able to commute by bus or train. Still in the process of correcting my credit from my previous mistake of running up my credit cards, I had to buy a hoopty (an older model car). But for a long time, it got me from point 'A' to point 'B' without much trouble. Whenever it would break down, I would remind myself that "God always looks after children and fools"; because I never stayed stranded on the road for any long periods of time. And keeping in mind that we didn't have cell phones then; I had to rely on strange passersby to stop to aide me with my car problems. I never had an incident where anyone tried to take advantage or harm me and I know that was God looking over me.

It seemed whenever I'd be on top of things, I'd relapse. During one remission period, I had decided to enroll in cosmetology school. After going to several hairshows with my puberty girlfriend, Gigi from California, I decided that I'd do hair. We grew up together in Saginaw and both left home after high school but have remained friends throughout the years. When she visited me in Newark and we attended the NY International Hair Show I was really impressed. Then later that summer, I visited her in Oakland, CA and we went to The Black & Gold Hair Show. So now I was going to cosmetology school in Rutherford, NJ in the evenings. It was a nice little hike from Newark but I was making it. I made it through the summer and fall and then I began to relapse. There were days when I cramped so badly that I would have to drive to work and school with a hot water bottle pressed on my stomach to relieve the pain while I drove on the freeway. By the time I made it to my destination, I would force myself to put on a front that all was well with me.

Although I was still taking the same medications, after some research, I decided to try the bayberry enema which I would purchase from a health store. I would boil the bayberry tea like substance and give myself an enema to relieve the pain and cleanse the colon. This seemed to be very effective initially. However, when I discussed this with my physician, he quickly recommended that I discontinue the use of the enema. I can't remember what his argument against this form of treatment was at that time. Whenever I would ask him why the relapses kept reoccurring (due to the fact that I followed all of his medical and nutrition regimens), he would say that it may be that I worry too much. He said I was always worrying about something; be it financial, professional or my personal life, etc. He also would tell me that I needed to learn how to say words like "no" and tell people "where to go". He said I was always trying to be too nice (people pleaser). I was holding in too much emotion inside and that was harmful to me. Today it's called "stress". I believe there was some (probably a lot) truth in what he was saying.

However, over the years I'm grateful that I have learned that it's not that I was holding in too much that bothered me—but it's the realization that everything is not always about me. Therefore, instead of an unnecessary confrontation with someone I must quickly access whether or not it's about me or if it's their own personal issue; which does not always warrant a reaction or response from me. No need for an 'one up' or 'last word'.

Aside from working and going to cosmetology school, I still harbored the desire to model. Although I never modeled as a professional, I had a great time doing local runway modeling at fashion shows. I was blessed to have worked with Jherald Walker, who was a very talented, young, African-American man that attended Parsons School of Fashion and Pratt School in N.Y. He lived near me and he would watch me come home everyday and liked the way I dressed. He was an aspiring dress designer so we became very close friends. Whenever I was preparing for a big event, he would design my outfit from head-to-toe. His sketch would also detail things such as jewelry and hairdo (or hat if appropriate). Then he would make the finished product. He was awesome. Most of my modeling work came from working with Jherald to show off his designs and I was loving every moment of it. The last piece he designed and made for me was in 2002. He made me a beautiful evening gown to wear to the newly elected Mayor Kwame Kilpatrick's Inaugural Ball. Sadly, Jherald passed away shortly after finishing my gown.

With my very hectic schedule during 1980/81, I no doubt began to relapse again. I was driving with the hot water bottle more often. Some nights as I was driving home from school, I'd have to pull over to the side of the road to throw up. I'm sure passersby thought I had had too much to drink but I was really, really sick. By the morning, I'd get up and start the ordeal all over again. The challenge for me was to make it through work and any other commitments I had for the day without seeming like there was anything wrong with me. I believe that because of these challenges that I faced on a daily basis is the reason for my low tolerance for people that come up with a million excuses why they can't make it. Especially when they are healthy people.

In the spring of 1981, I had gotten an assignment at the newly opened Medical/Denistry center which was across the street from where I lived. This was great. When I was feeling bad, I could come home for lunch and try to get myself back together before returning to work. In May of that same year, I was devastated with the loss of my little sister, Sandi. My mother and step-father had 2 younger daughters (Sandi—13 years younger than me and Tanya—15 years younger). Sandi, who had just turned 14, was at school and suffered from a brain aneurism which was fatal. That was a very hard time for me. I felt as if I had lost my own child. My teenage years were spent raising my 2 younger sisters and my niece. With both parents working full-time, I had to baby-sit for them. I resented this for years and swore that I would never have kids of my own. Now I was an emotional wreck. It probably would have done me some good to seek therapy for my loss but I did not. Instead, I ran out to California and stayed well over a month between L.A. and Oakland before returning back to Newark.

Summation:
More Tools

Being diagnosed with a chronic illness and having to change a job that you thought was a dream come true made me realize that I am definitely dispensable in the workplace. Therefore, I needed new mechanisms to help me deal with these events. I needed to be able to work on improving my health and not telling anyone of my condition for fear it might hinder my growth in the business world. I also needed to be able to be prepared to draw from my previous tools, if needed, to help me in making the right decisions to continue making it on my own without doing anyone or anything wrong. Discretion; courage; flexibility; and individuality were the tools I added on now:

<u>DISCRETION:</u> As a child, I always heard the expression, "don't let your right hand know what the left hand is doing". So it was no surprise to me that I chose to be secretive about my disorder towards friends and co-workers. As for my family, it was easier for me not to have them worrying about me or trying to convince me into returning home. My father had came to visit me while I was hospitalized the first time but he didn't fully understand what the disease was so once I was released from the hospital, he thought I was healed. Therefore, my secret was safe and to look at me, no one would know that I was suffering from a medical disorder. (Now that I am sharing with people about my

disorder, I'm getting the same response from most of them and if I hear it again, I just might SCREAM!!!) Their common response is: "You look so good." "You don't look sick." Well, I've put up a good front for 30 years. My disease has nothing to do with how I look (other than the occasional moon-face).

COURAGE: It took courage for me to go into New York and seek employment. Not knowing anything about NY other than what I'd seen on television or read about. Courage is what led me through the subways and streets of New York, without fear. I think when you're young, you tend to have more courage (maybe your boldness is born mostly out of naivety than anything else) to venture into the unknown. As you get older, you no longer feel the necessity to take such daring chances in life, so you tend to become more cautious with age (maturity).

FLEXIBILITY: I had to be open to keeping my options open. I couldn't be constrained to a timeframe. I had to learn how to multi-task early on so that more tasks could be completed within a certain window of time. This was the tool which enabled me to continue to work on my dreams of modeling; go to night school for an additional skill and maintain my job all at one time. Also, with my being an independent, single woman, I could jump up and move at any time, if needed.

INDIVIDUALITY: I had to be able to set my own standards. Set myself apart from others, to avoid being a follower or part of a clique. Especially if the clique was living the wrong lifestyle; I didn't feel the pressure of doing what everybody else was doing. During childhood, I was exposed to family members and friends living in the fast lane. Even though I never chose that lifestyle for myself; that exposure turned out to be to my advantage because it helped me in identifying the game before it even approached me. Running around in the subway and train stations in New York were real places where little naïve girls can easily become victims of hustlers.

MORALS & VALUES: One of the most important things my mother taught me in my younger years was the importance of morals and values. This is what gives you a strong foundation. When you know and understand the concepts of morals and values, you cannot go beneath a certain threshold. That's why when you hear a person say, "I hit rock bottom" and turned their life around; it is because of that foundation that was set in their life at an early age. That same foundation is set when you grow up with a church background. These same morals and values will not allow you to do wrong or misuse others for your own personal gain. That is why I chose my independence and worked hard to take care of myself. I realized that if I worked hard, I could buy my own things.

Chapter Three
Hi-Rise Robbery...
Gotta Go!!!!

After having lived in my apartment for almost six years, it was time for me to move on. With my long hours of working and traveling, I spent less and less time at home. Someone noticed my schedule and broke into my apartment one day while I was away. It was a frightening experience to walk up to my door and see that it had been left opened by an intruder. It really feels creepy to know that some mysterious person has been through your personal effects. Immediately I began making arrangements to move out. Because I had followed some good advice of a previous co-worker, I did have renters insurance so I wasn't hurt financially by the loss.

I had already planned to purchase a co-op prior to the break-in so I was able to make my move happen faster. Once I moved to Plainfield, I also followed the advise of my then boyfriend and began a new policy of not giving out my address to everyone I knew. As he reminded me, as much as I would be gone, there was no need for everyone to know where I lived. To this day, I am still the same about giving out my address.

By 1982, I was in remission and feeling great again. Each time that I would go into remission, I would subconsciously convince myself that I was cured. I would bounce back and continue all of the different quests that I was continuously involved in. Since I was living in Plainfield, I took on an assignment at Schwartz & Andolino Law Firm in Livingston and transferred my cosmetology credits from Rutherford to Somerset (which were closer to my home). I eventually settled for a manicurist license to shorten the timeframe of schooling. Now I was able to use my manicurist license to begin a part-time business for an additional income. I rented space at a local beauty salon and also a flea market where I did acrylic nails and tips on the weekends. With the additional monies, I was now able to work on getting my credit back on track.

I was feeling good, looking great and ready to start living again. During this year, I really took advantage of my good feeling. I spent a lot of time going to concerts (attended a fantastic tribute to Count Basie at Radio City Music Hall and also spent the 4th of July that year at my childhood idol's concert performance of the phenomenal Diana Ross). It really is a big thing when you can go to concerts or different events without the worry of being bothered with your symptoms. The first thing you have to do when you suffer from this kind of disease is to make a mental note of where the nearest restroom is to your seat; wherever you go. That alone is bothersome. But it has to be done. Since I have always been a very outgoing person, I would try not to miss certain events; i.e.; Essence Annual Awards, Ebony Fashion Shows, Music Festivals, etc. And at some of the events, I'd be embarrassed when I would have to go to the public restroom with my beautiful gown on to relieve myself. As time has gone on, it is now almost impossible to make plans in advance; because your good days are so limited that you don't want to pay for a ticket that you may be too ill to use.

CHAPTER FOUR
'FIXIN' TO GO AGAIN

I was pretty happy with my life in New Jersey with my close friends (which I am still close with today) and did not have any plans of leaving until I kept getting calls from friends that had moved out to Dallas. They were originally from Saginaw and had moved to Texas and really did a good job of building Texas up to be the best state anywhere. They talked about the fantastic weather, job opportunities and most importantly, the low cost of living. It started sounding good to me so after doing a little research, by the end of 1983, I was packing up to make another move. When I stepped off the plane in January 1984 (I had flew in from Michigan so I was draped in fur coat and hat, boots and a wool suit), it was in the mid 70's in Dallas. I had found my new home.

For those of you that have suffered with Crohn's will understand that it is very important to have your privacy. I had lived alone ever since the inception of this disease and now was living with someone for the first time. I had moved in with my uncle until I could find a job and an apartment. It was very embarrassing to me when I would go through my relapses. I would have to keep plenty of tissue and air freshener in the bathroom. If I were having a bad day, I may have to stay in the bathroom for over ½ hour at a time before coming out. I would be totally embarrassed if he had to go in after me. Even though he never said anything to me, I know it must have been out of love because I would leave a scent in the air that even I couldn't stand.

Again, with the assistance from a temporary agency, I was able to secure a job right away. As a matter of fact, I was hired in permanently with Blue Cross/ Blue Shield as a data entry operator. It had great medical benefits, of course. Since I had sold my old hoopty prior to leaving New Jersey, I was back to relying on mass transportation. I never had a problem taking public transportation. I think it is one of the best ways to learn your way around a new city; because you will have to transfer buses to get from point 'A' to point 'B' which will take you all over the city.

After only being at Blue Cross/Blue Shield for three months, my supervisor called me into her office to tell me how great she thought I was doing and that she thought I was overqualified for that particular job. I was beginning to get nervous, thinking she was about to let me go. But she said that she had a friend at Hunt Oil that was looking for an executive secretary for one of their vice presidents and that she had spoken to her friend about me. She set up an interview for me to meet with her friend. She swore me to secrecy not to tell my co-workers what she had done for me. A few days later, I met with her friend, along with the vice president that was hiring. We had lunch together and I was hired on the spot.

Within a few months of my relocation, I was settled into my own apartment, working as the Executive Secretary to the Vice President of Woodbine Management Company (which was a subsidiary of Hunt Oil Company). That was not only another great job opportunity for me but with a very impressive company. I was amazed by the history of the famous H. L. Hunt family. This was also a great experience because I was working for one of the wealthiest families in Dallas and when we had our grand opening for one of our new buildings in downtown Dallas ("The Founders Square)", the then Vice President of the U.S., George Bush, Sr., was our guest speaker. Because Dallas had already been the scene of a fatal politician's shooting years ago; everyone in our building had to go through the secret service screening prior to the event. As I can remember, they ran checks on our driver's license and whatever other inquiries they may have had at that time.

Because of my medical condition, I did seek out a physician once I settled in to Dallas. He ran his series of tests on me and gave me the same prescriptions I had taken in New Jersey. He also put me on an exercise program. I had to go to the medical center about 2 or 3 times a week to work out. Since I no longer had my manicuring side income, I took a part-time job at the local Montgomery Wards which was within walking distance of the medical center. That didn't last a full week. I never realized how much work retailers required of their employees and I couldn't hang.

Over the years, with my different jobs, I have been very fortunate to obtain more education and training through various company incentives. I would always take advantage of these opportunities. Once I was hired in at Hunt Oil, they sent me to a Lanier Word Processing class. This was in 1984 and at the time, word processing was taking over the electric typewriter (which was the most advancement towards technology for me).

My remission was holding out greatly and everything was going well for me. I had made new friends and was really enjoying being in Dallas. There were a few times during my commute to work when I had to seek public restrooms, but generally I was doing ok. This was probably the longest period of remission for me in a while. I'm not sure if it was due to the change of climate and atmosphere, but whatever it was, I was thanking God everyday. I spent an enormous amount of time on the bus. Not only commuting back and forth to work, but because my company provided me with free monthly bus passes, I would also use the pass on the weekend to do all of my shopping. To keep myself occupied during the rides, I always had a book in my hands. That way I didn't have to be bothered with small time chat with the neighbor sitting next to me, if I chose not to.

Having lived in northern states all of my life, it was refreshing and yet astonishing to me how integrated Dallas was. I knew that racism still existed, of course, but it was different than the northern racism. Up north, you'd be made to believe that you were accepted. In Texas, if you weren't accepted, you'd be told up front. No hypocritical "smiling in your face while stabbing you in the back." And I could appreciate that. So with life's experiences that you must go through as a test, it was finally my day of reckoning. It was in December 1985 while my boss was away on vacation that the office manager (a Caucasian female that I knew never cared for me) decided to let her true colors out. She began demanding me to do something and she just went on a tyrant. Before I knew it, she was coming towards me and yelling. There were other co-workers in the office at the time and I was infuriated by her behavior.

I didn't know how to act—so I reacted. In a spur of the moment, I jumped up and told her "where to stick the job." STUPID, STUPID, STUPID!!! I neither had the sense nor the tolerance to be calm, let her know that her behavior was unacceptable and I would report her to my boss upon his return. I didn't think far enough ahead to start looking for another job before walking out on this one; if I couldn't come to a resolution between her and myself. Oh no. I went off like a crazy woman and quit my secure job. I'd like to blame it on the emotional swings that I go through while on the medications…but I don't think that was it. It was pure stupidity on my part to leave. After learning about the situation upon his return, my boss phoned me at home to ask that I return to work so we could work things out. However, I told him that since things went down the way they did, I could never re-track what I said to the office manager, nor could she re-track what she had said to me. Therefore, I declined his offer to return.

Lesson learned—don't go off and leave a job without a back-up plan. Thank God, we learn from our mistakes—most of the time.

So here I am in the midst of the Christmas holiday season and unemployed. So as always, I went back to my old standby, Kelly Services. It only took one phone call before they sent me right over to Fidelity Investments in Las Colinas. They needed data entry operators for the 3rd shift. I started right away.

Chapter Five
Hey Girl...This is
a Man's World

❧

When I began my new temporary job at Fidelity, I never would have imagined that it would turn out to be a 20 year career for me. This was the first job I ever worked on the 3rd shift, so that in itself was an experience. At that time, Fidelity was in a hiring frenzy. More than half the people I worked with had began as a temporary employee and later hired on permanently. There may have been about 25 employees in my department. Our job was to input orders for mutual fund literature prospectuses for prospective and existing clients. The majority of the people in my department were like me, new to the world of investments.

In the beginning, I had no intention of staying there long. For me, it was just a temporary job to get me through to the next job. However, the company made it so easy for you to want to stay. Since we worked at nights (we usually began at 7 or 8pm), our lunch was well after mid-night. Therefore, most nights, lunch was brought in for us. They would bring in Grandy's dinners, Chinese, Pizza, etc. They would also bring in the largest, sweetest oranges for snacks. It was such a casual atmosphere that each person had a tape recorder or radio on their desk; ashtray for smokers and we would sit and listen to our music, while inputting data for 10 to 12 hours every night.

Overtime was unlimited, so we usually worked a lot of hours. There were so many smokers in our department that there was a constant cloud of smoke in the air. It had gotten so bad at one point that they eventually provided each desk with a new 'smokeless' ashtray. It ran by battery and was supposed to clear the smoke. That didn't last long. So they eventually banned the smoking in our work area and confined it to the cafeteria. No more smoking at the desk. At that time, they also took away our music.

After about a six week temporary run, I finally accepted a permanent position. I figured company benefits would not get any better than the ones they offered. And besides that, I was in my 30's and it was time for me to get serious and start looking at my future, as far as starting some kind of retirement savings plan. I had wasted 10 years in retirement savings so I needed to get serious. So on 2/10/86, I became a permanent fixture at Fidelity. I was about to embark on a career that was traditionally known as "A Man's World"; and to be frank—it was "A White Man's World." And in

Texas! But I was still in remission and back into my "I can do anything" frame of mind. So I was ready for the challenge to enter into an entirely new world of an industry that I knew very little about (except the basics which were covered in some of my college courses previously).

The first thing I had to do was to buy a car because there was no easy bus route at night from Dallas to Las Colinas. I purchased an older model Volkswagen Bug from a little old lady for $850 cash. The car was in good shape but I had never driven a stick before so I had to have someone teach me how to drive it. Initially, I did ok, until I was trying to get up a hill and stop. After rolling back down the hill with on-coming traffic coming towards me a few times, I became an expert.

Once I began permanently, I had no intentions of remaining a data entry operator. There were so many opportunities and since this was a growing company; I felt that it would be very easy for me to advance within the company. Most of my co-workers were African-American, Latino and some Asians. Most of the supervisors and work leaders were Caucasian and I didn't have a problem with that. It didn't take me long to notice that a lot of my co-workers were content with their positions and never discussed advancement opportunities within the company. There were a few that took full advantage of the opportunities available and went on to grow with the company in various other departments; but on the whole a large majority did not want to grow with the company and had that "who do they think they are" attitude towards the ones that tried to advance. Therefore, I knew that it would be best for me to stay to myself, excel at my job duties and try to learn as much as I could. I mean how long can you sit and key in repetitious information without your mind going idle?

By April/May 1986, I was promoted to the Remittance Department as a charter operator and my job was to process checks and bag the checks up for bank pickup. It wasn't until that time that I became aware of the multi-million dollars that we were taking in on a daily basis. Since I was the only person working on the 3rd shift in the new department, I had a lot of responsibilities but welcomed the challenge. After months of hard work and training a few co-workers how to do this job, I got my first reality check. Of course, one of them was promoted as the new work leader of the department. I insisted on changing to the day shift to avoid working under the person that I had just trained.

Now that I was working days, I set out to find a part-time evening job at American Airlines. I didn't take the job for the income. I took the job for the flight benefits. I worked as a part-time telemarketer and most of my payroll checks were minimal because I would fly for the cost of the taxes of a flight and it would be deducted from my paycheck. I became a regular bird. I would fly to California just to get my hair done or go shopping and return home later that evening.

During this period, I was able to attend a lot of events. AWED (a women's organization) held an all day workshop in New York one year and Oprah Winfrey was the guest speaker. I was able to attend the one-day event because my flight tickets were so inexpensive.

The flight benefits were a huge advantage during this period for me. I really missed having those benefits once I was no longer working for the airlines.

It was now 1989 and I was still doing okay medically. I was still taking the same medications and my remission was holding on well. My personal life was good socially and financially.

My stress level was doing okay, as well. I purchased a cute little two bedroom condo in Arlington and was enjoying remodeling it. Only this time, I was a little wiser. I was using the pay-as- you-go method to redecorate.

Since I loved working downtown Dallas, I was really excited when I saw a job posting a position for a customer service representative in the downtown investor center. Since leaving Hunt Oil, I missed the hustle and bustle of the downtown activity. Not only was it my desire to move into an investor center, but I also knew this would be the stepping-stone that I would need to go even farther within the company. I put together a very comprehensive package and set up an appointment at the Dallas office. The interview went exceptionally well. The following week, I received a call from the Dallas branch manager inquiring how long it would take me to find a replacement for my current position and be ready to transfer over. We agreed on a week's notice. I was told I'd be notified early the following week with the final details of the transfer into the new position.

In all of my excitement, I never saw it coming. An African-American in the investor center working face-to-face with the clients—in Dallas!! Well, it hit me like a brick upside the head when I received the call saying that they had changed the pre-requisites of the position and they were now looking for someone that was already licensed (stockbroker). He reiterated that he thought I was very qualified for the position and had no doubt that I could do the job, but it was out of his control. As a consolation, he said that he would notify personnel how well I had interviewed and wished me the best of luck. That's it. That's it? Oh, that's definitely not it!

I wrote to the Human Resource representative demanding a response, in writing, within so many days explaining to me why they had changed the pre-requisites of a job position which had already been posted. I also wanted to know if a new posting would be going up showing the change. Well, instead of responding to me in writing, a few days later I received a call from Human Resources saying that there just happened to be the same position opening in the same building that I currently worked in. In the few years that I had been with Fidelity, I had never even been inside the investor center downstairs. So I interviewed for the position with the branch manager and the following week was offered the position, with the stipulation that I had to take the Series 7 exam (licensing for stockbrokers) within 30 days. Okay! I'll take it!

Hence, this was a ground-breaker. I was the first African-American to work in the Las Colinas investor center. I was so proud of myself. This was an opportunity for me to learn more about the brokerage business first-hand. I'd be in the branch working with the sales staff, as well as the traders.

But hold up! Here comes a major slap in the face. The regional manager came into town to visit and immediately had contractors come in to build a wall around my desk area. Not just any kind of wall but my area was being encased with the blackest tinted glass that I have ever seen. To make sure that I wasn't seen, the encasing went almost up to the ceiling. I was totally offended. I was so offended that I refused to sit at my desk except for the times when I absolutely had to. I spent as much time as I could standing behind the front counter, greeting the clients. Initially, some of the regular clients seemed to be shocked to see me there. A few made some disparaging remarks but after a short period of time, they accepted me. Most of them instantly liked me. I had no problem acclimating to the new job responsibilities and except for that damn black cage, all was going well.

As promised, I took the exam by the 30 day deadline and failed it. By then I had proven to the manager that I could do the job so it was no longer a requirement.

Summation:
Additional Tools

As I said earlier, being born and raised in the north, I really needed a tool to help me deal with racism better. I had to learn how to handle it without harming myself in the process. Growing up during the years of the Civil Rights Movement, I had experienced the race riots in Detroit while on one of my annual summer vacation visits at my dad's. It was a very scary experience for me and I couldn't wait to return to Saginaw. My parents weren't involved in the movement so I had no real knowledge of what was going on in our immediate area but I did now that the southern states were not a place for me. As a matter of fact, when my family went to Georgia in the 60's, I refused to go with them. I stayed home with my grandmother. I remember telling them that I hoped they weren't returned home in the large picnic basket they had packed food in for their trip.

Now that I was living in the south, I felt that congeniality would be a good tool to help me deal with racism. I also needed to have faith.

<u>CONGENIALITY:</u> I found that if I presented myself with a pleasant personality, having a sincere concern for others and willing to listen with open ears, I'd go a long way. Once a person knows that you can be helpful, apathetic to their issues and have a sincere smile on your face; they are more than willing to give you a chance. If a person is not wooed by my friendly

personality, they probably just have issues beyond my concern.

<u>FAITH:</u>   My faith was a constant. I had to have faith to go through what I was dealing with. Not only the health situation, job changes and relocation to a new state; but it was faith that also helped me get through the acts of racism that I had encountered. Faith kept me from letting any negative forces set limitations on me.

CHAPTER SIX
HOW I LOST MY
BELLY BUTTON

◦⌘◦

The beginning of 1991 came in with a Blast! I was pregnant. In all of my life's dreams and goals, children had never been in the picture. So what was this? Here I am at the age of 35 with an unexpected pregnancy. This was definitely not part of my plans; an unmarried woman in a professional world having a baby. Not only was I embarrassed, but I felt that everything that I had been working towards was going to be stifled. After spending many days crying and praying, I finally decided that I could do it. I could be a single mom and continue in a professional world. So what's next? Well, unexpectedly during my first trimester while returning home from my annual night out at the Ebony Fashion Fair Show, I got very sick. By the time I made it home, I was bleeding. My doctor told me to get to the emergency room right away. The next day, I miscarried. I was very sad about the loss and cried for days afterwards. Even though my doctor had advised me to stay off from work for 6 weeks, I chose to return to work sooner. I needed to stay busy and keep my mind off of the miscarriage. When I met with my gastro doctor, he advised me that I shouldn't try going through a pregnancy again with all of the problems that I was having with IBD and I agreed.

Later that summer, I was back on track mentally and physically (so I thought). My father was having a heart by-pass and I was considering moving back closer to home by this time. I even went so far as to apply for a position in the Chicago branch. I didn't get the transfer. I was initially told that they didn't want to hire outside of Chicago due to the moving expenses. However, they did in fact hire an employee from Dallas for the Chicago position. Since I never got an interview, I guess I'll never know why I wasn't considered for the position. But I wasn't bitter. I guess it wasn't part of the master plan.

When you feel bad about things that are going on in your life, I have learned that it always helps to make yourself available to bring hope into others' lives. Therefore, I signed up to volunteer time in the "Adopt a School Program." One day each week, I would go to an elementary school and sit in the classroom with the young kids and help them with their school assignments. These were mostly Latino children that were struggling with the English language; because the majority of them were from homes where Spanish was their primary language. I enjoyed working with the children and really felt that I was doing something good.

By the end of the year, I began to relapse. The symptoms were worse than ever before. I didn't know if it was the stress, along with the miscarriage, but all of a sudden I was having sickness on an almost daily basis. My doctor immediately put me back on the Prednisone. He said if this didn't help, we would have to consider my going back into the hospital for possible surgery. The Prednisone gave me a temporary relief. In February, I had to go on a business trip to Memphis. Like always, I had to hide the fact from my colleagues that I was feeling horrible. I had been putting up a front for so long that it seemed natural for me. But this time the travel took a toll on me. To make things worse, upon return from Memphis, I had to go to a week long class at Dearborn Financial. I really didn't need to be going through a relapse at this time.

About a week or so after the class, I was in the restroom at work and passed out. I was rushed to the emergency room by one of my co-workers and hospitalized. I remained in the hospital for three days and by the middle of the following week, I was back to work. Medicated to the hilt; but I was back. I returned to work as if I had just recovered from a flu bug or something. There was no need to explain to anyone what I had been hospitalized for. Surely, if I can't discuss this with family, I didn't need to discuss it with co-workers. Also, on my personal side, I was back to attending friends' social events within a couple of weeks as if nothing ever happened.

By April, I was admitted into the emergency room again. I was in so much pain. I couldn't hold anything on my stomach and could not stop regurgitating. I was admitted again. All of my usual tests were performed while I was in the hospital. I was finally released to go home a week later. This time I was being treated with Flagyl and Prednisone. Hopefully, this would bring me back into remission soon. This relapse had been going on for some time now and my usual small frame of 110 pounds was going down.

In May, I was sent on another business trip to Ft. Lauderdale, FL. I didn't enjoy the trip as much as I would have liked because once I returned to my room each evening, I was trying to prepare myself physically and mentally for the next day's training class. Since on most of my business trips, I was usually the only African-American and sometimes, one of very few females; it wasn't too hard for me to disappear and not be missed during the after hour events. Once I returned home from the trip, I still was not feeling any better and within a week was having severe stomach cramps and very nauseated again. In addition, I was unable to defecate.

I was taking laxatives and stool softeners but they did not help.

By June, my weight had fallen below 100 pounds when I entered the hospital's emergency room. My doctor (Dr. Lagon) had run an extensive number of tests on me during my week long stay. When he came into my room with the results, he sat on the side of my bed and looked like he wanted to cry as he broke the news to me. I had a perforated ulcer (which was cancerous) and if I didn't have surgery immediately, it could burst and could be fatal. I had to make a decision right away.

I tried to maintain my composure when I phoned my mother to break the news to her. She immediately insisted on my coming home for the surgery. By her having worked at St. Luke's Hospital for so many years, she felt the best surgeon to perform this type of procedure was Dr. Dennis Boysen. As she began making arrangements for my hospitalization there; I began making arrangements with my surrogate family in Dallas. Darryl and his wife Sheila quickly made arrangements for his brother, Charlie to fly home with me. I was in almost a comatose state and could not travel alone. They also would take care of my condo while I was away. Two days later, after receiving my diagnoses, I was on my way home for surgery.

When I got off the plane, I was greeted by a host of shocked family members. From the looks on their faces, I could tell that they thought I was coming home to die. I was wheeled off the plane in a wheelchair, weighing 85 pounds and balled over in pain. On June 29, I was admitted to the hospital. Friends and family kept coming into my room but I did not notice they were there. I was in so much pain, I was delirious. For the next few days, prior to my surgery, we did a lot of praying. With all of the prayers from so many pastors in Saginaw coming to pray at my bedside, as well as family and friends, we prayed for healing.

On July 2, I had a gastric resection for a perforated duodenal ulcer (which was cancerous). In layman's terms, the doctors said I had to have almost half of my stomach removed. They said the outcome of the surgery was something of a miracle. It was like the cancer was isolated into a pouch in one spot and once they removed that section, the cancer was gone. No chemo-therapy or radiation required. The Power of Prayer! It is so awesome.

Now it was going to be a long road to recovery. I remained in the hospital for almost a month before being released. I was on morphine for the pain and could not eat anything by mouth for days. My family was no longer looking like they were going to lose me and that was a relief for them. It was never a doubt in my mind that I would be healed. As a matter of fact, all the while I was in the hospital, I had a great attitude for someone as sick as I was. My grandfather, who would come and sit with me everyday, had brought me some tapes by Rance Allen and I would play them over-and-over again, all day and night. I would pray for healing. I knew then that the materialistic things in my life didn't matter. I would easily turn over everything just to regain my health.

Once I was finally released to go home, I realized how great it was to have such a loving family to help me recuperate. Even Toby, the family dog, stayed at my bedside during my recovery. I was told that I had to take walks several times a day as therapy. So Toby and I would walk up and down the street several times a day. It was a long and painful process to recovery. Especially when you're used to being so active on a daily basis and now all you could do is lie around in the bed all day.

During recuperation time at home with my mother, I had a brief relapse and had to go back to the emergency room for an overnight stay. I had eaten something that I shouldn't have and had to have my stomach pumped. So I had to go back on the bland diet. But now I was feeling better and could at least hold food on my stomach again.

I remained in Saginaw recuperating until October. Upon return to Dallas, I was so grateful for my friends. They made sure I returned home to a clean home, with a hot, home-cooked meal waiting for me. Just knowing they were handling things back home for me was a huge relief. I had enough on my mind getting healed.

Once I returned to work, I immediately saw a big change. We had moved into a new location and the staff in the investor center had grown immensely. I had a lot of catching up to do. I had been out for so long. There were so many questions by co-workers about my medical condition. I simply told them that I had to have surgery which I didn't wish to discuss in details. I was feeling great and ready to get back to where I had left off.

When I returned to Dr. Lagon, he told me that because of the removal of part of my stomach, I'd do well to get back up to 100 pounds. He said I should just accept the fact that I wouldn't gain more than a few pounds. Yet each time I visited him for follow-up appointments, I was regaining my weight back. It was true; I could not eat much. This is when I began using a saucer for my plate. But I would eat maybe four or five times a day. I still eat the same way to this date. Little did I know then, this is the healthiest way to eat meals.

CHAPTER SEVEN
CHRISTMAS GIFT FRENZY

Since I had lived away from family for so many years, I probably tried to over-compensate with gifts at Christmas time. Every since I had left home in 1975, I would always try to make it home for Christmas to spend the holiday with my family. As the years went by and my financial situation improved, the more I was able to give. I saw this as passing on my blessings. Over the years, it was my belief that because I am such a generous and giving person, God always increased my blessings (or favor) because He knew I was self-less and would be there for others in need.

Well, this year, I realized how much I had spoiled my nieces and nephews. They were accustomed to my giving out great gifts. However, after being out on sick leave for almost half the year, this year I was doing good just to make it home for the holidays. I had little money to spend on gifts and just bought the kids little token gifts. Well, this didn't go over well with the kids. They wanted to know if "that's it?" I was so angry and disappointed with their reaction to my small gifts that right then and there I let them know that they would not have to worry about me giving them anything else. I told them that they were ungrateful little brats and that there were kids in the world that wished they had a gift. It was that year that I vowed never again to run around in the Christmas frenzy trying to buy gifts for family. Now don't get me wrong. If at any other time of the year I'd see something that I wanted to buy someone, I would. But no longer would I play Christmas with them.

But out of this unpleasant experience; came a new Christmas tradition for me. Tom Joyner, now a nationally-known radio personality, ran an annual Christmas campaign to sponsor a child at Christmas. Each morning he would read off a letter from an adoptive or foster child on air and you could either phone in to pledge all or part of the child's wish list. Then he would have a grand Christmas Party for the children to present the gifts to them. If you were unable to phone in a pledge in advance, you could just show up at the party with unwrapped toys and clothes for the children. I chose to do the ladder. It was such a fulfilling and touching experience just to see the faces of gratitude and pure elation on the faces of those kids.

CHAPTER EIGHT
AM I GOING BACKWARDS??

In 1993, my father was ill with his heart condition again so I was beginning the new year contemplating more seriously relocating closer to home. Since I had undergone such a serious surgery and the fact that my parents were getting older; I figured it would be more cost-efficient for me to go back home. While I was home for the holidays, I had met with the branch manager in our Birmingham, MI office. In all of my years in Michigan, I had never heard of Birmingham and had no idea where it was. Surprisingly, I was very impressed with the little quaint, up-scale suburb in Oakland County. The manager said they weren't hiring at the time, but would keep my name and resume on file for future reference.

Back in Dallas, I returned into my usual pattern. Working long, hard hours and spending time with my friends in my spare time. I was coming along well. My biggest obstacle was sleeping. After having been in the hospital for so long (where sleep is something you don't get much of due to the prodding, poking and medicating), I had a very hard time sleeping at night. But other than the lack of sleep, I was coming along well. To look at me, a person would never had known that I had just been delivered from a near-death situation.

By the end of January, our Regional VP was visiting the branch and he and I had a long conversation about my previous interview in Birmingham. Apparently, he was livid that the branch manager had even interviewed me; giving me some sort of false hope that they'd be hiring in the near future. He said because it was a new branch, they were fully staffed and had no plans of adding on more staff in the near future. For my inconvenience and being mislead, he said that there was a new office about to open in Woodmere Village, OH (a suburb of Cleveland). If I were interested, he could help secure me a position there. The branch would be open that April.

Immediately, I began doing research on Cleveland. My older sister lived in Akron, OH so I phoned her to find out as much as I could about the area. I began looking on-line for apartments (being careful to stay out of areas with check cashing stores in the neighborhood).

For the next few months, I had my hands full; looking for an apartment in Ohio, making arrangements with a property management company in Arlington to lease out my condo and finding a moving company. I also had to decide whether or not I would drive my car or have it towed. My sister decided to fly in from Akron and help me drive back. I was receiving a moving expense check and wanted to make sure that I could cover all expenses off of the check and not have to use any of my personal monies for the move.

On April 1, my friends had a 'going away party' for me at Steve Harvey's Comedy Club in Dallas. When I told Steve that I was celebrating my move to Cleveland, he had a huge laugh. He wanted to know, "why would you leave Dallas to go to Cleveland; are you crazy?" But I got the last laugh because it was the move that would change my life forever; a blessing that I could have only received in Ohio. Not saying that Cleveland was a great place to live. I never did like it during the five years that I lived there, but as I said before, it was part of the master plan and I had to go through it.

Once I got settled in to the new location and moved into my new apartment in Akron, I found myself looking for similarities to Dallas. There weren't any. Many cloudy, gray skies and yes, of course lots of snow. I had spent more time in Dallas (during my adult life) than I had lived anywhere else before. It felt as if I had left home for the first time all over again. But I looked at it as a good change. I had my health back and I was closer to home.

Even though the doctors that had performed my surgery months ago said they could no longer find any evidence of Crohn's Disease in me after the resection procedure was done, I was referred to a doctor at Cleveland Clinic to follow up with for an annual exam. I was feeling healthy and was ready to make my time in

Ohio work for me. With the medical nightmare behind me, I phoned my friend Darryl in Dallas to ask that he send me some clothing and art work from his African Store so I could start a side business in Akron. I soon opened up a booth at a local flea market in Akron and began making a nice side income for myself. I also had begun doing the expos and art fairs on the weekends.

Back in Dallas, my condo was being leased out but I wasn't making much extra income from it. It appeared that many months when I received my invoice from the property management, there would be some sort of repair bill attached for something. The condo was in great shape when I left it. Most of the appliances were new, the carpet was new and all of the walls were freshly painted so I didn't know whether the repairs were being manufactured on the invoice or not. But when you live so far from your property and not able to fly back and forth to check on it, you have to go with what is being told to you as fact. So I continued to hold on to the condo.

Everything was going smoothly now and I began to think about my purpose in life on a more spiritual level. I felt that there was a purpose for me and that is why my body healed. I began having serious thoughts about the possibility of sharing my life with a child who did not have anyone. So out of curiosity, I attended an adoption orientation meeting in Cleveland one evening. There, they showed video tapes on children that had grown up in the foster care system. They also gave statistics that were mind boggling. According to their information, African-American children were at an alarming rate in need of placement. I walked away from that meeting enlightened about the adoption versus foster care process. The visions of the children I had seen on the tape really saddened me. I didn't know if I could go through this process but I was glad that I was informed.

During that summer, I was diagnosed with having a hernia (as a result from my surgery). My stomach was pretty large for my body size. So I had to make arrangements to go in for a hernia repair surgery. To avoid taking time off from work, I made arrangements to have the surgery done during my vacation which was scheduled for the Thanksgiving weekend. Prior to leaving for Saginaw for the surgery, I began making phone calls to the radio stations in the Akron area to find out if they ran the same kind of Christmas campaigns that Tom Joyner held for the adoptive children. I was given the name of an African-American Adoption Agency, called Akiba which was located in Akron. I phoned them to find out what kind of Christmas gifts they needed and was told anything I could give would be welcomed. They were having their annual Christmas party for the kids the first weekend in December.

After I returned back to Akron from having my hernia surgery, I started making plans to prepare for the Akiba Christmas party. Shopping for the children made it more enjoyable and a lot less stressful. I just went into Walmart, filled a cart with toys for both boys and girls of all ages and dropped them off at Akiba. It gave me a great feeling to know that my gifts would mean so much to some children.

Now that I was in remission again, I was doing a lot better. I wasn't too exited about living in Ohio, but I worked a lot of expos within the state on the weekends and I also felt good enough to start traveling again. Although my credit had been repaired, I still continued to live below my means. I never wanted to over leverage myself in debt again. It was too easy to go over-board and too hard to come from under. Therefore, instead of looking to purchase another condo in the Cleveland area, I continued to rent. I had purchased my first brand new car (Toyota) prior to leaving Dallas so I had no large ticket items to be concerned with at that time.

I had been feeling great physically so I was quite surprised when on March 2, 1994, I had to call my sister to take me to the emergency room. The same previous symptoms were back again. All I could do was cry. I was in excruciating pain in the stomach area and could not stop regurgitating. I was admitted into the hospital and after many tests were run, I was told that I had a blockage from the previous resection surgery and they would have to repeat the same procedure again. I was scared to no end. I didn't want to go through that same painful surgery again, but I had no choice.

My family came in from Michigan to see me through the repeated surgery. The second time around was not a breeze. It was worse than the original surgery. I remained in the hospital this time until March 15 and released. Thankfully, I had an aunt from Detroit to volunteer to stay in Akron and nurse me back to health. I also had a nurse come in a few days a week. My recuperation was again slow and painful. And of course, I had to return later that year for a repeat hernia surgery.

After recovery from the last surgery, I was back to work and working long hours. As much time as I had to take off from work due to medical reasons, I felt guilty. Since I received four weeks vacation time each year, I usually would cash in at least one week and work. This not only allowed me to catch up on time missed, but also would show my loyalty towards the company.

We had a new branch manager the beginning of 1995 and during her first month, she had to have an emergency surgery and would be out for over a month. A lot of changes were being made at that time. We had a few of the sales staff transfer out of Ohio, or leave the company. We were very short staffed and I was working a lot of hours. I was feeling very healthy again and was able to work the long hours without incidence. Personally, I was enjoying the Akron/ Cleveland area about as much as I could—with what I had to work with. There were always training classes going on within the company which required me to travel which I always welcomed just to get out of Ohio for a few days. When there wasn't training classes, there was always another branch that needed someone to come help out for a few days or a week. So when an offer came for me to cover for a week in Raleigh-Durham, NC, I was all over it.

Once I returned from NC, I was preparing for my 40th birthday party. Since I had recuperated from two more surgeries within the past year and was feeling wonderful, I was ready to have a large celebration. So all of my long time friends (from all of the previous places I'd lived before) all flew in to Akron to celebrate my birthday with me. It was an outstanding event!

Not long after my 40th birthday, I began to look at where I was in life on a different level.

Here I am 40 years old; now a healthy, single woman with no children. I made a good living; I wasn't meeting anyone that I was interested in having a committed relationship with. It was this time that I began thinking about becoming a single parent. I didn't have to have a husband to become a mother. I would waver back-and-forth with these thoughts, off and on.

Summation:
More Tools Needed

The period of 1991 through 1995 really tested me. My previous tools helped me to sustain some of the issues going on but there were a shortage in areas that I had never been faced with or either tuned-out before. I have always been a praying person, but now I had to pray more than ever before. I didn't know if I knew how to pray in the dimension that was required of me. I needed help. I had major surgery coming on the heels of a miscarriage.

Another challenge that I had not considered was living so close to family after having been so far away from them for so many years. Now, I was only a short drive away. I turned to prayer, philanthropy, diplomacy and persistence during this period of my life.

<u>PRAYER:</u> Having such a major surgery was a very frightening ordeal and I had to pray for healing. In addition, the surgery not only makes significant physical changes in your body, but it also causes a lot of emotional feelings to surface that I could not deal with without the power of prayer. This is a tool that I will always treasure and will continue to work on growing in this area.

<u>PHILANTHROPY:</u> Coming out of such a horrific experience in my personal life, it gave me great joy to be able to focus on helping others. This I know I can always do. Even if I have nothing monetary to give; I

can give my time and to someone on the receiving end, will appreciate that more than anything.

DIPLOMACY: Having been away from family since 1975; it was an adjustment living within a short car ride away from them. I needed to be able to handle renewing my family ties. This is still an on-going process. Having been living away for so many years, (all of my adult life); I felt that they still looked at me as the child they once knew. Now that I had matured into a single, independent woman that returned home with an abundance of worldly experience, I had in fact changed accordingly. Not thinking I was better than anyone else, not a snob, just grown up.

With the secrecy of my disorder there were times when I'd visit or we'd travel together and I'd insist on getting a hotel room. This would create a problem. "Why can't you stay with us? You know how we do it. We'll sleep on palates and everyone will be together." Sometimes, reluctantly I'd give in but most times, I would come on a separate date and check into a hotel prior to joining the others. That way I could have my privacy. This also overflowed into the eating category. Having suffered from this medical problem for so long, I had learned how to control my symptoms by not eating. Therefore, I would eat just enough to keep from starving in order not to have the symptoms flair up at an inappropriate time. And of course, unbeknownst to them my reason for not eating, some family members would see it as my not liking what they cooked or how they cooked.

PERSISTENCE: Although I had gone through hell medically, I never gave up on becoming a licensed stockbroker. I had received my Series 63 license years earlier, and now I had finally got the big one. The Series 7 exam would allow me to go further in my career.

Chapter Nine
The Homestudy Process

Legacy of an Adopted Child

Once there were two women who never knew each other; one you do not remember, the other you call Mother.

Two different lives shared to make your one; one becomes your guiding star, the other became your sun.

The first one gave you life and the second taught you to live it; the first gave you the need to love, the second was there to give it.

(Taken from Legacy of an Adopted Child...Author Unknown)

With the new promotion and raise, I was excited and looking forward to getting ready for Christmas. As I had been doing since moving to Akron, I was already planning on what I'd buy for the children at Akiba this year. To my surprise, one of the adoption supervisors at Akiba phoned me to meet with her just before the holidays to discuss my volunteering to help out at the upcoming Christmas Party. However, during our meeting, she kept trying to convince me how great a parent she felt that I would be for one of these children and hoped I'd consider adoption. Before I knew it, I was back at the adoption orientation meeting at Akiba.

The adoption regulations vary from state-to-state. In Ohio, if you are adopting from a state agency (such as Akiba), you have to go through the homestudy process. This is a very long and comprehensive process that the agency conducts to confirm that you are eligible to become a parent. The issue of being single was once a hindrance, but now that there is such a need for home placement for these children, it is no longer a major factor. They run an investigation on your history (credit, criminal records, etc.) and interview friends, family, and employers. You have to go through medical exams (which I passed with no problem) and they assign a social worker to do the periodic surprise visits to your home. The process was long but uneventful.

Once I had successfully completed the homestudy process, it was time to meet the children. It was, and still is, disturbing to me some of the statistics that I read on adoption. There is an astronomical number of African-American kids that are in need of home placement. What disturbed me even more was the statistic which showed that the dark-skinned little boys were the least requested for adoption. Therefore, my caseworker seemed shocked when I informed her that my pre-requisite was to find the darkest, nappy-headed little boy I could find.

My initial visit with my son was all I needed. The agency had ran a match and the little two year old boy was what I had asked for. The caseworker informed me that she had more children she wanted me to meet before making my final decision, but I didn't need to meet anyone else. It wasn't as if I was shopping for a pair of shoes. My intent was to provide a loving home to a child and this child needed a loving home. Therefore, we proceeded to the next steps.

Going through the states for adoption, requires that you make so many visitations with the child before actually placing him with you. My son had been in a foster home since birth. He and three other foster kids lived in a home with a Caucasian family. The foster-mother had a teenaged daughter that my son was very attached to. I could tell by her interactions with the children that she was in all probability the primary caregiver for these children. There was about a 35 mile ride from my job to their home. I would leave work everyday and drive over for my pre-arranged visits. This went on for several weeks before I could finally take him off their premises. I would pick him up and take him to a public place (I wasn't allowed to take him to my home yet). We'd go to the playground or McDonald's to spend a couple of hours together. Initially, he would scream crying when I would try to take him away from their home. Now he was screaming crying when I had to return him. It would break my heart.

That summer, I had decided to host our family reunion in Akron. With approval from the agency, I was finally able to keep him for an entire weekend so he could attend the family festivities. The family fell in love with him immediately. He just fit right in. My nephews, which were his age, bonded with him right away. They are stair-steps and are still very close. The one thing that I did notice that weekend was the fact that he could put away some food. It was like he had tasted many of the foods for the first time and he was enjoying it.

Later that summer, we went through the legal process at the courthouse and we were officially mother and son. It was hurtful to me that none of my family was there to share that momentum event with us but my son and I rejoiced. We went home and prayed together. And we continue to pray together. We were blessings to each other.

After taking him to Saginaw to have him 'Christened', we had family and friends come from all over to celebrate in his 'welcome to the family' celebration. We were so blessed. He was welcomed into the family and the label adoption has never been put upon him by either side of the family.

As I continue my gift giving at Christmas to the children in need, it has been a pleasure for me to see that my son has also been a blessing in this area as well. From our first Christmas together, he has always helped me in picking out toys for the kids. This is my way of teaching him the value of unselfishness and sharing.

Chapter Ten
Full Circle —
The Return Home

I had my first emergency as a single-working mom the beginning of the year. My son, an otherwise healthy child, had the chicken-pox. Since my sister, who lived in Akron also, had to work just as I did; I had to pack my son up and make the drive from Akron to Saginaw. My mother would keep him and nurse him back to health and I wouldn't have to miss work. Well, that was the plan. As fate would have it, once he was cured from the chicken-pox, I returned to Saginaw to pick him up. While sitting at my nephew's basketball game the following morning, I had a horrific itch all over my body. It was so bad that I went to the emergency room to see what was wrong. Yes, even though I had had the chicken-pox as a child, I had them again. And let me tell you; there is nothing worse than a 40 year old woman covered from head-to-toe in Aveeno oatmeal around the clock for days. The healing process was long and miserable. The blotches on my skin never fully went away but I eventually healed enough to return back to work.

Once getting over the chicken-pox fiasco, all else was falling into place for us. I was still in remission and we were moving along. Being that I had been single and accustomed to doing things when and how I wanted to, now I had to make major changes. I feel that there was a huge advantage in my waiting to become a mother later in life. By that time, I had done just as much as I wanted to do. I was established financially and now I didn't feel that I would be missing out on anything by devoting myself to becoming a mother. I still could do a lot of things; I just made them family-oriented events. I was enjoying this new found lifestyle.

I still had to make the occasional business trips, but I was always able to get a family member to come and baby-sit for me while I was away. That is probably why during the spring of 1998 when I received a call to come to Birmingham, MI to help out, I was excited to go. There was a new branch manager there (which I had worked with in Ohio) and he knew that I was interested in relocating to Michigan. After about the second day helping out at the branch, I was offered a promotion and relocation package. I spent the rest of the week looking for a new place for me and my son to live in Michigan. I was excited for the opportunity to raise my son near my family.

Almost immediately, I was being prepped to go into sales. I had worked most of my career in customer service and really enjoyed what I was doing. And I was making a decent income. I wasn't in sales; however, a large percentage of my client interactions would turn into large sales opportunities. I was aware that I had a talent for turning service interactions into sales interactions. But I lacked the confidence of working in sales because of my conservative nature. I needed to know exactly how much I was earning. I was afraid of working in sales when my income would be largely based on commissions. However, my new manager saw that quality in me and within a few months, I was studying for my insurance licenses. Once I was fully licensed, I was ready to step out on faith again.

With much apprehension and concern, I eventually entered into a sales position. I did not just enter into it; I roared in with the tenacity of a bull. I never realized before how competitive I was. It was a continuous goal for me to be ranked in the highest category for all sales interactions. I worked this position as if it were my own private business. Being the sole African-American in my new position (for our company in Michigan), made me feel pressured to be noticed as a great performer. In order for me to do that would require my doing something different than my colleagues to bring in business.

Therefore, I began to go outside of the office to bring in new business. It would be nothing for me to meet a prospective client at their place of business or a designated common meeting place. By the end of 1999, to look the role of a successful financial planner, I had purchased a new Jaguar. I would drive to Lansing, Flint, Bay City and any other town there may be potential business. I had begun scheduling so many appointments in the Saginaw/Bay City area that I started using a local hotel in the area as my meeting place. At one point, I was referring to the hotel as 'my office in Saginaw'; because I was going there so often.

I was on a roll. I was surprised how great the job was going and wondering what took me so long to do this. My sales performance had almost immediately advanced into a six-figure position. I was in the top rankings and loving every minute of it. My disorder was still in remission so I was able to work the many hours which were required of me to be successful in this position. I was working on an average ten hours a day. I was usually the only person in the office to schedule weekend appointments; in order to accommodate clients that due to their work schedules were unable to come in during our regular business hours. If I weren't holding an appointment on Saturdays, I would be there to catch up on paperwork or make phone calls. I was amazed at how much business I was doing. I was generating multi-million dollars in business on a weekly basis. The many hours spent at work were paying off and as a result, I have successfully received the Achievers Award as well as the Chairman's Award over the years due to my hard work.

Because of my grueling work schedule, I made sure that when I wasn't working; my time was my son's time. I made sure that we'd take at least one big trip together each year. We'd go to a different state and do something that would be an educational adventure for him as well. I also made sure to free up my work schedule to attend whatever school programs he'd have. Personally, when I wasn't working, my life had turned into my being a chauffer/ chaperone for my son but I wasn't complaining.

Now that my financial situation was better than ever; I was trying to do all of the right things. I was maximizing my 401k contributions, as well as adding to IRA and UTMA (college savings for my son) accounts. Because of my illness, I honestly believe that I would over-compensate in what I was spending on clothes in an effort to cover up how awful I was feeling inside. Therefore, I would spend $2,000 to $3000 for an outfit and think nothing of it. And of course, I had to have a hat to complete the outfit. I would take the outfit or a swatch of fabric to the millinery store and have a hat customized to match my outfit. I have paid as much as $800 for one hat. My justification for this bad behavior was the fact that I wasn't running up credit cards. I was paying cash. I would convince myself that because I was making all of the other right financial decisions (saving and investing), that I was justified to spend as much as I wanted on clothes. Eventually, I regained my senses and discontinued that madness.

In 2001, I had my annual colonoscopy and endiscopy. The tests results showed that the Crohn's Disease had become active again. At that time, I was put on Colozal and Prednisone. The pain and nausea was not a major fact yet. But the frequency for the bowel movements had increased so much that it caused rectal bleeding. For that, he prescribed me some Cort enemas to relieve the pain. There was little else that could be done at the time.

So now I'm back in the office and making my road trips as if everything is normal. Because of the mood swings from the medications I was on, some days I'd sit at my desk and all of a sudden, I'd be overwhelmed with sadness and start crying. I'd run to the restroom so no one could see me crying. In an attempt not to let my disorder interfere with work, I continued working the long hours. The biggest inconvenience was that there was no restroom directly in our office so I spent a lot of time running down the hall to the restroom. To kill the bad odor, I would light a cigarette in my stall. Since it was a public restroom I figured no one would know it was me lighting up.

Over the next few years, I had several more hospitalizations dealing with my disease. However, it was always the same thing; back to the Prednisone. By now they had changed me over to Asacol, replacing the Alzulphadine. I had such a concern that I had been on the ladder for so many years that I didn't feel it was effective. Also, I had a concern that prolonged use of the drug could negatively affect other organs in my body (i.e. the kidney, liver, etc.). I also remained on my bland diet. I made every attempt to keep my stress level down during the times of my relapses, which was getting harder to do.

By the end of 2004 and the beginning of 2005, I was having more severe symptoms and was concerned that during my annual exams there were no new treatments being recommended. I felt as if I was going through the motions of having these tests while my colon would deteriorate to the point where it could no longer function at all. These symptoms were really taking a toll on me at work. It had gotten to a point where I'd have to increasingly disappear from my sit-down consultations with clients in order to run to the restroom. I may disappear for 10-15 minutes at a time. I'd always return to the appointment feeling guilty as I made up an excuse for my absence. Because no one else in my office knew what I was going through, I couldn't ask them to cover for me. It wasn't until 2005, after a brief hospitalization, that I finally broke down and informed my manager of my disease. I didn't go into any details or try to explain the disease to him. I didn't feel comfortable talking about my symptoms. I just wanted to let him know why I was feeling sick so frequently.

In February 2006, as I went for my annual tests, I was informed by my physician that I would have to be admitted into the hospital immediately. I was diagnosed with Exacerbated Crohn's. Also, as a result from the Crohn's, inflammation was now going into my hip joints, causing me to have arthritis. Now I was also having severe pain in my hips. I had already been on the maximum medications for some time now so I was prescribed Remicade. (This is an infusion treatment for severe Crohn's patients. Initially, I would go to the hospital once a month for treatments; now I only have to go once every two months.)

After a week in the hospital, I was finally released to go home. During my hospitalization, I had a couple of consultations with a team of surgeons that recommended surgery for me.

They felt that because my colon could no longer function in the capacity of allowing me to fully control my bowels, that I should have the colon removed. They explained that this surgery would not be a cure—but would improve my quality of life. Instead of going to the restroom ten times a day, I would decrease that to maybe four or five times a day. Now that I was home, I decided to phone the surgeon in Saginaw that had performed my previous surgery for a second opinion.

When I met with Dr. Boysen and his team, he also agreed that I should have surgery. After a lengthy discussion of the ilesolomy and colectomy procedures, he recommended that I consider having the colectomy surgery. He said that it could reduce my symptoms, however, it was not a cure. He suggested that if my condition remained uncontrollable through medical management that I should strongly consider the colectomy. Because no physician has ever told me that the surgery is a cure—and also due to the fact that they tell me the disease will re-occur after several years—I still have not chosen to have the surgery. If it's not going to cure me and if it comes back; what's the next step? I'll be less an organ with the same disease.

Because of my deteriorated condition, my doctor placed me on an indefinite sick leave while I began undergoing the Remicade treatments. While dealing with my illness and contemplating surgery, I was under a tremendous amount of stress. Also, being on the maximum amount of meds, including pain and mood swing pills, I spent most of my days crying. Since I had kept this disorder a secret for so long, I was having a hard time trying to convey to others what I was going through.

After only being out on sick leave for a few weeks, I stopped in my office one day to have some papers faxed to human resources when to my surprise—I no longer had an office. All of my pictures, personal belongings, and files were gone. In shock, I hurried out of the office and returned home. Once I was in the privacy of my home, I balled. I cried because I felt that I had been replaced that quickly and no one even bothered to notify me. Now the shock had manifested into anger and I returned to the office demanding that all of my personal belongings be given to me right then. With the manager being out of the office, I was told that my belongs had been put in storage because they were uncertain when I'd be returning to work. Whether I was being paranoid or insecure, I demanded that my belongings be placed in my car. Therefore, two of my colleagues carried out the boxes to my car as I continued crying in disbelief. With all of the medical stress I was under; now I was worried about my job security. Once my manager returned, he notified me that my things were put into storage because we were planning on moving into a new location in a few months and he didn't know when I'd be returning to work.

Because I was on an indefinite leave of absence, it really floored me when after my second month of being out on short-term disability; my insurance carrier informed me that I would no longer receive payment. Just like that. I went from making six figures to $0 within two months. I was in a panic. The insurance carrier had determined that even though I was taking infusion treatments and still under the care of my physician, I could still perform my work duties. They recommended that I put on a 'depend' and ask for extended bathroom breaks, as needed. Even after my doctor sent numerous documentation stating my condition would not allow me to perform my duties, they would not reverse their decision. For the next few weeks, I spent each day making phone calls to the insurance carrier, breaking down crying during our conversations, trying to get their decision reversed. It seemed as if every time I spoke with them, they were requesting more documentation from me. I was continuously getting copies from various doctors to confirm my condition and sending them to the insurance company in hopes of a reversal. After about a couple of months, I felt I was going crazy and decided to hire an attorney.

I knew that with my condition, I would not be able to perform any work duties outside of my home. I was getting more and more depressed. I could not return to work in my condition and I was not receiving any income. I was still having a hard time talking about my symptoms and the disorder to others. During a conversation with one of our regional managers, I broke down crying. I attempted to explain to her what I was going through medically, as well as mentally since I was no longer receiving pay. She recommended that I consider seeing a psychiatrist due to the fact that I was having such a hard time discussing my disorder. At first I was offended by her suggestion. But after a couple of days contemplating her recommendation, I decided that it couldn't hurt me. So I scheduled an appointment to meet with a therapist to discuss what I was going through.

Once I began undergoing treatment for depression with a therapist, it did become easier for me to discuss my disorder with others. At least I was no longer breaking down crying. However, I was still stressed out and depressed due to the dealings with the insurance carrier. I had also filed for Social Security Disability during this time. Once I filed a claim with social security, I was immediately informed that the original claims are usually rejected so I should be prepared to appeal. And that is exactly what happened. Once I began the appeal process, I was informed that there would be at least a two year wait just to receive a hearing date.

Needless to say, my depression deepened as the months went by and I had no income coming in. I had the financial responsibility of two households (the home I lived in and a condo which was on the market to sale). On top of that, in order to maintain my insurance policies, I now had to mail in the premiums because there were no paychecks for them to deduct from. I felt my world was caving in. I would try to force myself on some days to act as if everything was normal but those days were decreasing more and more. My medical condition was worsening as the stress and depression was overwhelming me. I was going through a mental breakdown. I would sink into a self-pity state on some days and just spend the entire day in bed. My symptoms were not improving but getting worse and I found it difficult to even leave my house.

Because I was in the financial business, I was fortunate that I had taken the advice that I'd been giving to my clients for years. That advice was to always have at least six months income saved for an emergency. Well, that came in very handy during this time. But once the six months came to an end, I realized that six months income is not enough for an emergency fund. One year is probably a better target; because when there's nothing coming in, those six months seems to fly by. Especially when your medical condition does not allow you to return to work.

Because I had taken out a separate disability income insurance policy years earlier, I phoned that carrier to see if I could start receiving benefits. Because I had already been off from work for over six months, I now qualified to receive their benefits. It was only a fraction of what I was accustomed to making but at least it was something. It still baffles me how one insurance carrier could approve me, while the other continued to deny my benefits based on information from the same medical reports.

Almost a year later, after countless hours of praying and listening to spiritual tapes, I finally began coming out of my state of mental madness. Once I was able to finally step out of myself long enough to look at myself, I realized that I didn't like this picture. I had never been a weak person, but I had failed myself and my son. I had to pray for strength to get my mind back. I had to make a choice between making a large income and struggling with the pain and embarrassment of my symptoms (which were uncontrollable); or begin preparing to start a new way of living and take a large cut in income. I decided on the ladder.

It does not seem like it, but it has been almost a year since I've been out of work with my illness. I have spent the better part of this time inside my house. Because of my symptoms, I lack the confidence of being out in public, unless it is necessary. As much as I loved attending church on a regular basis, I had the difficult task of attempting to explain to my pastor of my frequent absence from services and what I have been dealing with. This has been hard on my son as well, but thanks to a supportive family, he has been able to take a few trips over this past year with them. I am trying not to let his life be effected by my confinement.

Not only has writing this book been cathartic for me, it has also been the one thing that has helped me keep my sanity by giving me something to do with all of this time on my hands. Being a person that has worked for over 30 years, it is part of my nature to get up at 5am to begin my day. Now I have something to look forward to. Getting this book out is important to me because I know that there are thousands of sufferers that are going through the same ordeal that I am going through.

My future is still unclear at this time. I have an appointment with a specialist at the Cleveland Clinic the end of February that I am looking forward to. I am hoping that we can incorporate natural healing in with my medical management program. I plan on spending the next few months researching various natural healing resources since the medicines does not seem to be working. The surgery would be absolutely my final chose; if all else fails.

As far as work, I know that I can no longer work in a traditional office environment, so I plan on looking to do something that will allow me to work from my home. I consider myself very fortunate to have gone through all of the experiences that I have been through over the years; as well as the good income I was able to earn. However, I realize now that the quality of life is much more important to me. Therefore, I am willing to earn less now if it means that I can reduce my stress level in an effort to improve my health.

I also hope that this book will be the beginning of my becoming a voice for the Crohn's and Colitis sufferers that are going through the same ordeal that I am dealing with. Not only here in the U.S., but also in other countries, there are thousands of sufferers which are forced to go through the economic hardship because although their symptoms are severe, they are being refused benefits because the insurance carriers, as well as Social Security Disability does not see Irritable Bowel Disorders as the chronic disease that it is.

Summation:
Tools To Sustain Me

Being out on sick leave without pay while suffering from a chronic disorder and depression put a different perspective on life for me. With the knowledge and experience that I have amassed over the years, I'd be better served using those skills working for myself. This time has also made me realize the importance to continue to have some savings set aside for emergency situations. The tools I plan to incorporate into my life going forward will be self-preservation; planning and advocacy.

SELF-PRESERVATION: The first thing I realized when my income was discontinued was that I had no one to go to for financial help. That is why I am so grateful that I had the insight to have some savings. I have always been a giving person, but I realize now that I will have to change my source of giving from monetary to giving my time or skills. I can't allow myself and my son to go through the economic hardship again. I am also talking to my son about this experience in hopes that he will concentrate more on how he can begin his own business versus working for someone else.

PLANNING: Due to the unforeseen, sudden drop in income, I realize how important it is for me to continue my financial planning so that I do not enter into retirement penniless. With careful planning and budgeting, I feel that I can get through this economic hardship. If necessary, I'm sure I could open a boutique with the items in my closet. I will continue doing research for sources of home businesses. I am not looking for one of the 'get rich quick' schemes that I see so many advertisements for. I am just looking to maintain what I have and can be happy with that.

ADVOCACY: I plan to continue researching the various Crohn's/Colitis websites to discuss with other sufferers the ordeals they are going through with regard to receiving insurance and disability benefits. I have sent emails to two of the senators in my state concerning the Patient's Bill of Rights (or lack thereof). Now I plan on spending more time bringing these concerns to the attention of someone who cares.

About the Author

Toni Whitley, a single mom, currently lives in Auburn Hills, MI. Having spent her adult years in Newark, NJ; Dallas, TX; and Akron, OH, she has obtained various licenses and certifications over the years. As a fully licensed stockbroker, she has worked in the financial investments industry for over 20 years. Since relocating to MI in 1998, she has been actively involved as a member of the Auburn Hills Chamber of Commerce Program Committee; member of the Birmingham Chamber of Commerce; member of Inforum (formerly Women's Economic Club) Volunteer Committee and a member of The Boys & Girls Club of SE Michigan Advisory Committee.

Printed in the United States
92743LV00001B/105/A

9 781425 996598